Defend Your Life V

Defend Your Life

Vitamin D and Cancer

Susan Rex Ryan

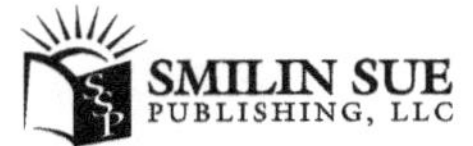

SMILIN SUE PUBLISHING, LLC

DISCLAIMER

The purchaser or reader of this book hereby acknowledges receiving notice of this DISCLAIMER. The author and SMILIN SUE PUBLISHING, LLC, publisher of this book, are not engaged in providing medical care or services, and the information presented in this book is in no way intended as medical advice or as a substitute for medical counseling. The information in this book is not intended to diagnose or treat any medical or physical condition or problem. If medical, professional, or other expert assistance is needed or required by the reader of this book, please seek the services of a competent expert. This book is based upon information taken from sources believed to be reliable. Although reasonable caution has been taken in compiling the information contained herein, this book may not contain the best or latest information and, in fact, may contain mistakes. The reader should use this book only as a general guide. The opinions expressed in this book are not to be relied upon as statements of fact. Anyone who reads or purchases this book, or any vitamin, mineral, or supplement mentioned in this book, acknowledge that they are relying upon their own investigation and not on any statements or opinions expressed herein, and are making their own independent decisions after discussions with their doctor or other medical professional. This book is sold without representation or warranty of any kind, express or implied, and the author and SMILIN SUE PUBLISHING, LLC are not liable or responsible to any person or entity for direct or indirect loss, damage, or injury caused or allegedly caused by information contained in this book.

Published in January 2024 by Smilin Sue Publishing, LLC.
smilinsuepubs.com
ISBN: 979-8-8620158-1-2

Book design by BookWise Design.
Cover source images by CI Photos, Shutterstock.

Dedication

To my dear Mom.

CONTENTS

INTRODUCTION

Cancer is common throughout the world. As an advocate of acquiring and maintaining an optimal level of vitamin D, I felt compelled to delve into the medical literature to better understand cancer and how it might be prevented or treated with optimal vitamin D3 supplementation. One thing is certain: there is an association between cancer and vitamin D status. *Defend Your Life V* provides several viewpoints for you, the reader:

The initial part addresses the fundamentals of vitamin D, including its various sources as well as its biochemical partners. Furthermore, the comprehensive testing chapter provides information including laboratory reference ranges of partners and substances associated with vitamin D.

Part II provides an overview of cancer including vitamin D's anti-cancer properties. Science— as I describe it in easy-to-understand language— indicates that vitamin D has a direct synergy with the prevention and treatment of cancer.

The second part of this book also addresses some of the most prevalent types of cancer including specific gene mutations that are related to specific cancers.

The popular Vitamin D Wellness Protocol comprises the third part of *Defend Your Life V.* This document describes how, by supplementing daily with vitamin D3 and two nutritional partners, you may optimally increase your vitamin D levels to boost your immune system. In other words, you can pursue how to decrease your risk of cancer as well as treat early-stage cancers. Tens of thousands of individuals have followed the Protocol, many of whom report achieving a healthier way of life.

I sincerely hope you find *Defend Your Life V* informative and useful. For our new readers, welcome to the amazing world of vitamin D!

~Susan Rex Ryan

PART I

Vitamin D Overview

1

VITAMIN D BASICS

Almost two decades ago, the words "vitamin D" were rarely uttered by the general population. Today "vitamin D" is almost a household word.

Despite its recent popularity, the concept of vitamin D has been around since ancient times. For example, Hippocrates, the father of modern medicine, used sunlight exposure to treat a type of tuberculosis.

More than a thousand years later, rickets, a disease characterized by soft and disfigured bones, emerged in Europe. Caused by vitamin D deficiency, this malady was initially documented in England in 1650. During the nineteenth century scientists began understanding the positive effect of ultraviolet B (UVB) sunlight on treating rickets. By the early twentieth century solariums were popular across the globe to treat diseases including rickets, tuberculosis, and rheumatism.

We discuss vitamin D and its significant connection to sunlight in the next chapter.

Now let's look at vitamin D basics. We know that vitamin D is technically a steroid hormone, produced by our bodies when we: expose our skin to UVB light; consume large quantities of fatty fish or vitamin D-fortified foods; or take a vitamin D3 supplement.

Unless you bask daily in UVB rays under the optimal conditions stated in Chapter 2, consume immense amounts of wild-caught fatty fish, or follow the daily Vitamin D Wellness Protocol included in this book, you might not have optimal levels of vitamin D that may decrease your risk of developing an array of medical conditions including cancer.

Many people—across generations and geographic locations—suffer from deficient vitamin

D levels because their lifestyles do not usually include vitamin-D-rich foods, unprotected sunbathing, or taking the proper supplements.

- A study published in *The Journal of the American Osteopathic Association* found high vitamin D deficiency prevalence worldwide. Two osteopathic doctors conducted a comprehensive review of vitamin D including its physiology, deficiency risk factors, diagnosis, and treatment. They found that about one billion people globally, or nearly fifteen percent of the world's population, have a vitamin D level of less than 30 ng/mL, well below the optimal level of 100 ng/mL (250 nmol/L).

Symptoms of low vitamin D include a host of common complaints such as muscle weakness, fatigue, bone pain, and chronic back pain, as well as susceptibility to contagious illnesses such as influenza. Vitamin D deficiency is easy to diagnose by having a simple blood test (Chapter 4) and to treat by taking three over-the-counter supplements daily.

Let's understand the basic process of vitamin D in the body. Our health is controlled and maintained by trillions of cells, the smallest units in the human body. The body's organs comprise millions of cells. Cells contain components called receptors that control what vitamins, minerals, hormones, and other substances (medications, free radicals, etc.) can enter or depart a cell.

Vitamin D receptors (VDR) receive and, in some cases, produce activated vitamin D. VDR are present from head to toe: in our brains, hair follicles, eyes, and skin as well as in, *inter alia*, our cardiovascular, endocrine, gastrointestinal, immune, musculoskeletal, nephrological, neurological, reproductive, and respiratory systems.

The most natural way to obtain vitamin D is from moderate exposure to UVB rays from the sun. When your skin absorbs UVB rays, your body interfaces with a chemical called 7-dehydrocholesterol and produces **initial** vitamin D (cholecalciferol). Alternative sources for vitamin D are cholecalciferol from over-the-counter supplements and limited foods.

It is interesting to note that cholecalciferol is included as an "essential medicine" in the World Health Organization's (WHO) List of Essential Medicines (EML). The EML "contains the medications considered to be the most effective and safe to meet the most important needs in a health system."

Once cholecalciferol is produced in the skin

cells, it enters the blood stream and travels to the liver. The liver processes—by hydroxylation—vitamin D into **circulating** vitamin D (calcidiol or 25-hydroxyvitamin D).

Circulating vitamin D travels along two distinct paths. First, the kidneys convert calcidiol into **activated** vitamin (calcitriol or 1,25-dihydroxyvitamin 2D). Activated vitamin D interacts with the parathyroid glands to maintain calcium blood levels.

Second, if circulating vitamin D remains in your bloodstream after calcium levels are maintained, the liver converts the leftover circulating vitamin D into activated vitamin D. The "excess" activated vitamin D travels in the blood to your tissues and cells and attaches to VDRs to perform functions essential to improved health including:

- Regulate gene expression.
- Reduce inflammation.
- Regulate cell differentiation, proliferation, and natural death (apoptosis).

These mechanisms of action are vital to protecting you from developing a wide array of medical conditions including allergies, autoimmune disorders, *cancer*, and osteoporosis.

How Safe is Vitamin D Supplementation?

Vitamin D toxicity is rare. As you have learned, vitamin D3 supplementation mimics the production of cholecalciferol in your body when UVB rays strike your skin. Scientific studies indicate that our bodies can naturally absorb at least 20,000 IUs from daily exposure to UVB rays to make enough vitamin D to protect us from most illnesses. I take 20,000 IUs daily to thwart contagious illness and maintain my overall health. Chapter 6 elaborates on how effective optimal vitamin D is to bolster the immune system in order to prevent cancer development.

Furthermore, a 2019 study in Ohio reported that, after seven years of over 4,700 psychiatric patients supplementing with vitamin D3 (either 5,000 or 10,000 IU a day), there were no issues with calcium and parathyroid levels. "Due to disease concerns, a few patients agreed" to supplement with 20,000 to 50,000 IU daily! The researchers concluded in the *Journal of Steroid Biochemistry and Molecular Biology* that "long-term supplementation with vitamin D3 in doses ranging from 5,000 to 50,000 IU a day appears to be safe." Therefore, a daily vitamin D3 supplementation of about 10,000-20,000 IU, as specified in the Vitamin D Wellness Protocol, is safe for most people.

Please note that persons who suffer from kidney and/or liver disease, or hyperparathyroidism, should consult a medical practitioner before taking vitamin D supplements. In addition, folks who are using cardiac glycosides or thiazide diuretics should check with their health care provider prior to using supplemental vitamin D.

Concluding Thoughts

Vitamin D is a steroid that is produced when cholecalciferol is in the body. Sources of cholecalciferol are UVB light, a limited number of foods, and over-the-counter supplements. Cholecalciferol is recognized by the WHO as an essential medicine under "Vitamins and Minerals."

Too much vitamin D in the body is rare. Nonetheless, the safest method of controlling your vitamin D3 supplementation is to monitor through blood testing your circulating vitamin D and calcium levels at least every six months until you have achieved a vitamin D status that you wish to maintain.

In the next chapter we address sources of vitamin D.

2

SOURCES OF VITAMIN D

The most natural source of vitamin D is expo-sure from the sun's ultraviolet B (UVB) light. The sun has provided its light including UVB rays as long as we have inhabited the earth. People originally lived and worked outdoors. They wore little, if any, clothing—and they lived near the equator, the closest distance to the sun.

Fast forward to the Industrial Revolution in the nineteenth century, two twentieth-century world wars, vast technological advances, and global economic markets. Today people live and work indoors. They commute and travel by enclosed conveyances. Air conditioning has become widely used at workplaces and in homes. These lifestyles have contributed to vitamin D deficiency.

Let's briefly review a decades-old campaign launched by the cosmetic industry. Seeking additional revenue, the cosmetic industry endeavored to market its products as not only beauty but "health" aids. In the 1970s, the cosmetic business reportedly began funding medical schools' dermatology departments with the intent to influence the American Medical Association (AMA) to educate the public about the dangers of sunlight. In 1989, the AMA issued a warning that caused millions to purchase and apply sunscreen and sunblock products. Well, you know the rest. The sunscreen business totals in the billions of U.S. dollars, and the sun scare continues today as does the prevalence of vitamin D deficiency.

Outdoor UVB Light

We do not need to hide our skin from the sun. The body possesses an inherent mechanism to produce vitamin D from the sun. The skin can produce about 20,000 IU of "intake" vitamin D a day depending upon several situational factors. After the body acquires enough D (usually about

20 minutes of ideal UVB exposure), the skin's safety mechanism turns off the initial production of vitamin D. Moderate exposure to the sun is healthy.

A varying number of factors affect the degree of UVB sun rays absorbed by our bodies to produce vitamin D including:

- **Geographic location**. Location is paramount to making vitamin D in your skin. The closer to the equator (lower latitudes), the higher the altitude, the better opportunity to acquire vitamin D-rich sunlight.

- **Time of day**. The higher the sun is in the sky, the better it is to obtain vitamin D from the sun. The hours of 10:00 AM to 2:00 PM local time are the best times to get vitamin D from direct sunlight. If your shadow is shorter than your height, you are in a potential vitamin D-producing window.

- **Season**. Many medical studies have demonstrated seasonal effects on vitamin D levels. The sun shines the longest period during the summer and the shortest timeframe during the winter.

- *Cloud cover.* An azure sky is highly preferable to cloud cover. UVB light is decreased by about 50 percent when penetrating cloud cover.

- *Air quality.* An adverse product of industrial civilization is ozone pollution, which absorbs UVB sun rays before they can reach your skin.

- *Age.* The older one is, the more challenging it is to obtain and maintain optimal vitamin D levels from sunlight. As people age, the concentration of the vitamin D precursor (7-dehydrocholesterol) in the skin decreases.

- **Weight**. Overweight and obese people have difficulty producing optimal vitamin D. As vitamin D is fat-soluble, the body's fat cells absorb this essential nutrient, decreasing its availability to the organs, tissues, and cells.

- *Skin pigmentation.* Melanin, the pigment in your skin, absorbs UVB rays. The darker your skin color, the more difficult it is to produce vitamin D in your skin. People with darker skin may require up to 10 times the sun exposure that light-skinned people need to produce vitamin D. African Americans have staggering rates of low vitamin D and accompanying incidences of medical conditions associated with vitamin D deficiency.

- ***Glass windows.*** Sunning by a glass window or door may feel soothing but it will not help you make vitamin D. Glass eliminates at least 95 per cent of UVB light.

- ***Sunscreen and cosmetics.*** The marriage of cosmetics and sun protection factors (SPF) will reduce the ability for skin to make vitamin D. The application of either product to your skin most likely will block UVB sunlight.

- ***Clothing.*** We are encouraged by public health to "cover up" in the sun. The more clothing we wear in the sun, the less vitamin D is produced in our skin. However, due to the risk of skin cancer, it is better to rely on taking vitamin D3 supplements.

Indoor UVB Light

Optimal conditions for producing vitamin D from the sun are dependent on a few elements. Some factors we can control, and others we cannot. So, what about using indoor sources of UVB light to produce vitamin D in our skin? For almost a century, UVB lamps have been used to treat some medical conditions.

Decades later, tanning beds became popular. People tend to frequent tanning facilities to look better, e.g., sport a tan during the winter. However, can the use of tanning beds increase vitamin D levels? The answer is "it depends." Having toured tanning salons, I found that most beds do not use UVB light. Ultraviolet A lights are the most common bulbs in tanning beds, but they do not stimulate vitamin D production. If you are using a tanning facility, ask specifically for a bed that only provides UVB light. (Do not be surprised if the facility does not have one.)

Using indoor UVB light is an individual choice. Personally, I have not been inclined to utilize indoor tanning. I opt for highly limited, outdoor UVB exposure and oral vitamin D3 (and K2) supplementation.

Food

Many Western diets are not rich in fatty fish caught in the wild. Foods that naturally contain vitamin D include salmon, mackerel, sardines, and cod liver oil. (However, cod liver oil contains a large amount of vitamin A, potentially disrupting vitamin D's processing. Please see Chapter 3.)

A number of foods are enriched with vitamin D, or cholecalciferol. Common vitamin D-fortified foods in the United States and the United Kingdom are milk, cereals, and fruit juices but they only contain small amounts of vitamin D. Enriched foods most likely will not effectively treat a vitamin D deficiency because large quantities of these foods would need to be consumed daily. For example, you would need to drink ten eight-ounce glasses of vitamin D-fortified milk daily to obtain merely 1,000 IU of vitamin D.

Vitamin D3 Supplementation

The most practical and effective treatment of vitamin D deficiency is to take a soft gel or liquid drop containing vitamin D3, in accordance with the Vitamin D Wellness Protocol addressed later in this book. Quality vitamin D3 supplements are readily available online or over the counter in retail stores.

The one truly effective vitamin D form is called vitamin D3 or cholecalciferol. Activated vitamin D3 is the bioidentical substance that our bodies recognize to perform essential health functions that include strengthening bones to decrease the risk of developing cancer, auto-immune diseases, and other serious medical conditions.

For decades, a less effective form called vitamin D2, or ergocalciferol, has been used in supplements as well as food and beverage fortification. Vitamin D2 contains synthetic compounds that are chemically altered and not well recognized by the body. Despite these facts, vitamin D2 can still be found in enriched foods and beverages as well as multi-vitamins and other supplements.

When selecting a vitamin D3 supplement, please carefully read the ingredient labels on vitamin supplements and fortified food and beverages to ensure you are buying D3—the "real" vitamin D! (Please note that people who have kidney or liver issues should consult their healthcare provider prior to taking vitamin D3.)

Beware of Prescription Vitamin D

Misperceptions about treating vitamin D deficiency still abound among medical practitioners and their patients. When treating patients for almost any medical condition, many conventional medical professionals "automatically" write prescriptions—the perceived "holy grail" for effective treatment. In turn, patients usually salute smartly by taking the prescription. However, in the case of treating vitamin D deficiency, beware of prescriptions.

At least in the United States, vitamin D deficiency is often treated with a *prescription* for "vitamin D." Guess what? The prescribed vitamin D usually contains the less effective form of vitamin D2 (ergocalciferol) that I addressed above. Patients usually take one *prescribed* 50,000 international units (IU) capsule a week, for about eight to twelve weeks. Most patients, however, are completely unaware that prescribed vitamin D2 comprises synthetic compounds that are chemically altered and not well recognized by the body. In my opinion taking a vitamin D2 *prescription* is like trying to fit a square peg into a round hole; the square peg simply does not fit! Prescribed vitamin D2 most likely will not significantly improve your levels. Therefore, your vitamin D deficiency will not be effectively treated. You most likely will not feel better and will be wasting your time and money.

Vitamin D3 Soft Gels and Liquids Are Better Absorbed

Vitamin D is dissolved in fat. Therefore, vitamin D3 supplements in soft gel or liquid form are absorbed better than chalky tablets or chewable, fructose-laden pills. The best time to take your vitamin D3 supplement is right after your breakfast. Healthy fats, including olive oil, egg yolks, and avocado, will facilitate the absorption of vitamin D3 supplements in your body.

Concluding Thoughts

Vitamin D3 supplementation is easy, effective, and inexpensive. In the next chapter you will see other nutrients that work closely with vitamin D3.

3

VITAMIN D'S PARTNERS

Vitamin D does not function alone in the body. Other vitamins and minerals interact as cofactors with activated vitamin D and perform the essential functions explained in Chapter 1. Fat-soluble vitamin K2 facilitates fat-soluble vitamins A and D's functions. The minerals calcium, magnesium, phosphorus, zinc, and boron also team with vitamin D.

Carefully read this chapter. The fact that specific vitamins and minerals function effectively with vitamin D does not mean that you should begin (or modify) taking supplements of these nutrients without consulting your health care practitioner. Please also consider that many of these nutrients can be obtained from your diet.

Vitamin A

The functions of vitamins A and D comprise the foundation of our health, regulating genetic activity that causes cells to make proteins required by water-soluble vitamins and minerals. Vitamin A deficiency is rare since common animal and plant foods contain this nutrient. Therefore, vitamin A supplementation is usually unnecessary.

A note of caution—when cod liver oil or retinol supplements such as retinyl acetate and retinyl palmitate are consumed on a regular basis, vitamin A toxicity may occur. Excess vitamin A in the body causes havoc because it prevents vitamin D from influencing the genetic activity described above. Vitamin A supplementation may obviate the wonderful benefits of vitamin D. Please be careful!

Vitamin K2

Vitamins K2 and D partner to build and maintain strong bones and teeth as well as fight cardio-vascular disease. Vitamin D's functions include regulating calcium absorption in the intestines to maintain bones and dental health. However, once calcium enters the blood stream, vitamin D relinquishes control of the mineral's destination to a less-known nutrient called vitamin K2—one of the Vitamin D Wellness Protocol trio—that moves calcium out of the arteries and into the bones and teeth.

Let's look at vitamin K2 and how it complements vitamin D. Like vitamins A and D, vitamin K belongs to a family of fat-soluble nutrients. Two distinct forms of vitamin K offer medical value: phylloquinone and menaquinone.

Phylloquinone or vitamin K1 is present in all green plants that acquire energy from sunlight. Green leafy vegetables including spinach, kale, collard greens, broccoli, and Brussels sprouts abound with vitamin K1. Clotting blood is primarily vitamin K1's life-saving benefit. Vitamin K1 constantly recycles in the body, so deficiency is rare.

Menaquinone or vitamin K2 differs greatly from K1. First, there are two forms of vitamin K2: menaquinone-4 (MK-4) found in *grass-fed* animal protein including meat, egg yolk, butter, some cheeses, and calf's liver. A more potent form of menaquinone, called vitamin K2 (MK-7), is abundant in a fermented soybean called natto.

Health benefits of optimal vitamin K2 levels include potential prevention of osteoporosis, arterial plaque, and dental cavities. Vitamin K2 moves calcium to the bones and teeth, as well as sweeps calcium from soft tissue lining such as the arteries. Specifically, vitamin K2 activates proteins (osteocalcin and MGP [matrix gla protein]), which are produced by vitamin D that facilitate moving calcium to where it belongs: the bones and teeth.

Low vitamin K2 levels, however, are common and may pose health risks. First, vitamin K2 receptors need regular replenishment as they are not recycled in the body. Second, the vitamin's natural sources are lacking in most diets. Owing to the reliance on industrial farming in many parts of the world, many people are low in vitamin K2. When insufficient vitamin K2 is in the blood stream, calcium can linger along arterial pathways potentially causing calcification, the process whereby calcium deposits form plaque accumulating in the cardiovascular system.

Supplementing with optimal vitamin D3 and K2 balances calcium metabolism. The concept of "balance" is important: one can enjoy optimal vitamin D levels but unknowingly have a vitamin K2 deficiency, a potential recipe for the development of cardiovascular disease. Unless you ingest *grass-fed* animal products or soy-laden natto on a regular basis, consider taking a daily K2 supplement that does not contain soy products. (For example, soy can interfere with thyroid medication.) Some experts recommend a daily dose between 90 and 120 mcg. WARNING: Some anticoagulant medications (blood thinners such as warfarin) block the action of vitamin K. If you are taking any blood thinning medication, please check with your health care professional before adding *any form of vitamin K* to your body.

Calcium

The essential mineral calcium is the best known of vitamin D's partners. Vitamin D regulates calcium's absorption in the intestines so it can contribute to bone and dental health.

Calcium deficiency tends to be uncommon as most Western diets contain sufficient calcium including dairy products, leafy green vegetables, and fish products. Calcium supplementation, however, remains a topic of debate within the medical community. While calcium is essential to the bones and teeth, this mineral can linger throughout the body, potentially causing calcification in soft tissue including the kidneys and cardiovascular system.

If you are taking a calcium supplement, you may want to reconsider. Since understanding the danger of calcification of soft tissues, I have not taken a calcium supplement because my serum calcium level is within normal range. Furthermore, I consume a daily vitamin K2 supplement to increase the likelihood that the calcium in my body is moved from the bloodstream to my bones and teeth.

Magnesium

The mineral magnesium is a member of the Vitamin D Wellness Protocol trio, which includes vitamins D3 and K2. Magnesium is essential to vitamin D's metabolism and absorption. An abundance of medical literature indicates that magnesium is one of the most important elements in maintaining good health. Its benefits include energy production, protection of the nervous system, improvement of muscle function, and a decrease in cardiovascular disease risk. Low magnesium levels may impair the conversion of circulating vitamin D to the activated form, denying your body vitamin D's amazing health benefits.

In today's world of fast food and pharmaceutical drugs, magnesium deficiency is common. Many diets lack natural sources of magnesium including green leafy vegetables, legumes, seeds, and nuts. Furthermore, prolific use of prescription drugs including antibiotics, proton pump inhibitors, and osteoporosis medications contribute to depletion of the body's magnesium levels. A daily magnesium supplement of at least 400 mg may boost your levels of this important mineral.

Phosphorus

Phosphorus (phosphate) is a mineral that interacts with activated vitamin D and parathyroid hormones to help maintain the balance of calcium. A wide variety of foods such as beef, chicken, eggs, seafood, legumes, nuts, grains, and dairy products contain ample amounts of phosphorus. An imbalance of phosphorus is rare except for persons with excess or extremely low blood calcium or kidney disorders. Unless ordered by a health care practitioner, phosphorus supplementation is not recommended.

Zinc

The essential mineral zinc works with activated vitamin D to bolster the immune system and influences healthy cell function. Zinc is commonly found in shellfish, red meats, beans, poultry, and nuts. Although zinc deficiency is rare, some people choose to supplement about 50 mg per day.

Boron

The trace mineral boron is essential to activate vitamin D's metabolism as well as the breakdown of calcium and magnesium. Boron is contained in fruits, vegetables, seeds, nuts, and other foods produced in plants. Deficiency of boron is rare as its sources are common in most diets. Some people choose to supplement boron but for most people it is unnecessary.

Concluding Thoughts

Vitamin D functions in concert with fat-soluble vitamins A and K2 as well as several minerals. To reap the health benefits of vitamin D, you should be aware of its biochemical partners, specifically vitamin K2 and magnesium, which are included in the Vitamin D Wellness Protocol in Chapter 13.

The next chapter addresses how to test each vitamin D partner as well as the parathyroid hormone.

4

VITAMIN D-RELATED TESTING

Testing your vitamin D level is paramount to achieving and maintaining safe optimal status. In addition, testing specific vitamin D partners or related biochemicals may be a good idea depending on your individual situation. Remember that vitamin D and its cofactors must be *balanced* to be effective.

Except where noted, the words "testing" and "test" mean blood is collected in your medical professional's office, local laboratory, or at home, and fasting prior to the test is not required unless noted in this chapter. Reference ranges of biochemicals vary from laboratory to laboratory so please use the numbers here only as a general guide. As always, I recommend undergoing testing under the care of your health care professional.

Vitamin D

Your first vitamin D test establishes your vitamin D3 baseline. The gold standard test for vitamin D3 is called **25(OH)D** or 25-hydroxyvitamin D where your available, or circulating, vitamin D3 (calcidiol) in the bloodstream is measured. The optimal range is equal to, or greater than, 100 ng/mL (250 nmol/L).

Another vitamin D test is called 1,25(OH)2D or 1,25-dihydroxyvitamin 2D where your activated vitamin D (calcitriol) is measured. This test is *not* the preferred test by vitamin D experts for these reasons: a) the biological half-life of calcitriol is shorter than calcidiol and b) the test is less accurate because the 1,25(OH)2D is influenced by the parathyroid hormone (PTH) as well as other hormones. Ensure the 25(OH)D, *not* the 1,25(OH)2D, test is ordered.

Calcium

Calcium is absorbed in the intestines through the action of vitamin D. A more-than-optimal vitamin D3 level may cause too much calcium in soft tissues and organs. So, it would be a good idea to test your serum calcium, which measures the total calcium in your blood. If **serum calcium** level is more than 10.9 mg/dL, then your parathyroid hormone should be tested.

Ionized calcium is the free, most active form of calcium. You must fast for the ionized calcium test, which should be taken if excess calcium or PTH is a suspected issue. The normal rage of ionized calcium is a level between 4.64 and 5.28 mg/dL. Low ionized calcium may indicate, *inter alia*, a vitamin D deficiency and/or low parathyroid hormone (hypoparathyroidism); abnormally high ionized calcium may suggest excess calcium and/or an overactive parathyroid gland (hyperparathyroidism).

Another method to ascertain calcium status, including the amount of calcification of the coronary arteries, is to undergo a CT (pronounced "cat") scan for your cardiac calcium. The name of the test is **"CT coronary artery calcium (CAC)" scoring** or something similar. Valid for up to five years and unknown to most of the public, the

CAC test is easy, fast, and non-invasive, and can be scheduled at your local radiology diagnostics center. The amount of radiation exposure is about equivalent to a mammogram, and no contrast dye is required.

The encouraging news is that the American Heart Association recommended the CAC test in its November 2018 cholesterol guidelines for determining cardiac calcium risk status and the need for statins for people aged 40 to 75 years. At the time of this writing, however, many health insurance plans do not cover the cost of this test. However, the test fee (usually less than US$200) is well worth the money. This test may save your, or a loved one's, life!

Vitamin K2

Vitamin K2 partners with vitamin D to move calcium out of the blood stream, soft tissues, and organs and into the bones and teeth. There is no generally available test to measure directly forms of vitamin K. However, a CAC test may provide insight into the effectiveness of vitamin K2 intake in your cardiovascular system. In other words, if your CAC score, serum calcium, and/or ionized calcium are low, your consumption of vitamin K2 probably is effective. If your CAC score, serum calcium, and/or ionized calcium are high, then your parathyroid hormone should be tested.

Parathyroid Hormone

Nestled behind the thyroid gland, four tiny parathyroid glands in your neck play an important role in your body: they regulate calcium. When calcium levels are too low, the glands release **parathyroid hormone (PTH)** to restore the *calcium* to its normal range. Conversely, when calcium levels rise, the parathyroid glands stop releasing PTH, potentially causing a range of symptoms including kidney stones and bone pain.

Three forms of PTH are assayed in this test for which *fasting is required*. The reference ranges are: N-terminal: 8 to 24 pg/mL; C-terminal: 50 to 330 pg/mL; and intact molecule: 10 to 65 pg/mL. If any of your PTH forms are out-of-range, then explore further options with your doctor. For example, high PTH (hyperparathyroidism) could be directly related to a low vitamin D status.

Magnesium

The mineral magnesium plays an important role in absorption of vitamin D and calcium. The two most common magnesium tests are called serum magnesium and RBC magnesium. **Serum magnesium** is often ordered by health care professionals and evaluates the amount of magnesium in the bloodstream. The "normal" optimal range for the serum magnesium test is 1.7 to 2.2 mg/dL.

The **RBC magnesium** test, however, is preferred, owing to its accuracy. Most of the magnesium in the body is absorbed in the cells; this test measures the magnesium in the RBC or "red blood cells." According to Dr. Carolyn Dean, a renowned magnesium expert, the optimal range of the RBC magnesium test is 6.0 to 6.5 mg/dL.

Phosphorus

Absorbed in the intestines, the mineral **phosphorus** interacts with vitamin D, calcium, and PTH. The **serum phosphorus/phosphate** test measures the amount of inorganic phosphate in the blood; urine testing is also available. Phosphorus deficiencies are associated, *inter alia*, with malabsorption, excess calcium, uncontrolled diabetes, and kidney disorders. The "normal" reference range for serum phosphorus/phosphate is 2.8 to 4.5 mg/dL.

Zinc

A cofactor of vitamin D, the mineral *zinc* can be measured by taking a plasma (not serum) blood test called "**zinc**." (Zinc is challenging to detect in blood serum as it is only distributed in trace amounts to the cells.) Zinc also can be tested using a urine test or hair analysis. Zinc deficiency affects approximately two billion people across the globe. Low zinc is associated, *inter alia*, with gut health issues, autism, and mental health challenges. The "normal" reference range for the plasma zinc test is 10.0 to 17.0 µmol/L.

Boron

Boron is a little-known element that is one of vitamin D's partners. While it is not typical to supplement with **boron**, some people do, and blood or urine testing may be in order.

Vitamin A

Fasting is required for the **vitamin A** test that measures retinol, the animal form of vitamin A. Deficiency in vitamin A is rare in the developed world. Nonetheless, a low level may indicate malabsorption of this vitamin D partner. On the other hand, high vitamin A may suggest, *inter alia*, consumption of excess cod liver oil, which can cause unpleasant symptoms, including liver damage, bone pain, and severe drowsiness. The reference range of vitamin A for adults is 38 to 98 μg/dL.

Concluding Thoughts

Nature's *balance* of vitamin D and its cofactors works in unison. For most people, testing vitamin D3—the 25(OH)D test—and serum calcium every six months is optimal to monitor your Vitamin D Wellness levels. In some cases, an out-of-range measurement can lead to more tests. With that said, it is usually unnecessary to run the gamut of the tests addressed in this chapter unless ordered by your doctor. And, as we see, much of the available testing is related to balancing calcium–a vital mineral that commands "a check and balance" to ensure optimal health!

Part II is where we learn about cancer cells, their behavior, and how vitamin D can decrease the risk of developing cancer and potentially treat some early-stage cancers.

Vitamin D and Cancer

5

A BRIEF INTRODUCTION TO CANCER

The subtitle of this book is "Vitamin D and Cancer." You have reviewed the basics of vitamin D in the initial part of *Defend Your Life V.* The second part of this book explains how cancer behaves and vitamin D affects the process. The third part offers a simple routine on how to raise your vitamin D levels to decrease your risk of cancer.

We are familiar with the word "cancer" but what does it really mean? In fact, the C-word is one of the most dreaded words in any language. However, if I asked, "What is cancer?" to two dozen individuals, I would likely receive twenty-four different responses. Although many people understand that cancer is not contagious, they are unsure of what cancer really encompasses.

Cancer occurs when our cells go on a mutiny from healthy cells. Cancer is a *genetic* disease, which is caused by genetic mutations that incite cells to multiply at an uncontrolled state (*cell proliferation*), engage in *cell differentiation,* and wreak havoc by disallowing natural cell death (*apoptosis*).

An Ancient Disease

Cancer has long been known in medicine, dating back to about 3000 BC. The origin of the word "cancer" came later, by the "father of medicine," Greek physician Hippocrates (460-370 BC). Hippocrates used the words *carcinoses* and *carcinoma* to describe cancer's crab-like tenacles that wrap around healthy cells as well as DNA. Spreading its fearsome tentacles around healthy cells, cancer has probably been killing humans as long as we have occupied this planet.

Main Types of Cancer

The medical community divides cancer into four main types, depending on <u>where</u> *the disease begins.*

Carcinoma, the most common of cancers, begins in the skin or the tissue that covers the surface of internal organs. Carcinomas usually form solid tumors. Examples of carcinomas include breast cancer, colorectal cancer, lung cancer, and prostate cancer.

Sarcoma, an aggressive form of cancer, starts in the tissues that support and connect within the body including muscles, fat, nerves, tendons, joints, lymph vessels, blood vessels, cartilage, or bone.

Leukemia is a cancer of the blood that turns healthy blood cells into cancer cells and causes them to grow uncontrollably.

Lymphoma begins in the lymphatic system, a network of vessels and glands that help fight infection. The two main types of this cancer are Hodgkin's and non-Hodgkin's lymphoma.

Risk Factors for Cancer

Two categories of cancer risk factors include *innate gene mutations* and *acquired gene mutations.* If you were born with innate gene mutations, e.g.,

your parents each carried cancer genetic mutations, your risk of developing cancer is higher than
for people who do not have these inherited cancer
gene mutations.

Innate gene mutations may cause cancers
such as breast, colorectal, and ovarian. Having
innate, or inherited, cancer gene mutations does
not predispose you to cancer. However, you have a
higher risk than persons with only acquired gene
mutations from environmental factors. You can
find "Geek Speak" boxes for DNA gene mutations
associated with cancer risk factors throughout
Part II.

Another category of cancer risk factors can be
called environmental, *acquired* gene mutations.
Acquired gene mutations may increase cancer risk
by experiencing:

- first- and second-hand smoke (including
  tobacco and other smoking materials)
- alcohol consumption
- air pollution (including wildfire smoke and
  motor vehicle exhaust)
- industrial and household chemicals (including dry cleaning)
- processed food diet
- sedentary lifestyle
- aging

- radiation
- some viruses such as hepatitis B and C
- inflammation.

I believe that another acquired cancer risk factor is low vitamin D. You will not find this risk stated in most, if not all, public literature. However, scientific literature includes studies about vitamin D status and its role in preventing and treating some early-stage cancers.

Normal and Cancer Cell Development

The human body comprises trillions of cells. Healthy and cancerous cells each behave rather differently. Some examples include:

- Every day some normal cells grow old and die a natural death (*apoptosis*), only to be replaced by new, healthy cells. Cancer development cells are neither repaired nor replaced.

- Normal cells reach maturity before they die naturally, which is called *differentiation.* Malignant cells do not mature because they are undifferentiated.

- Cells that are normal stop growing when there are enough to perform their functions. Cancer cells grow uncontrollably; this process is referred to as *proliferation.*

- Normal cells respond to signals from other cells. Malignant cells ignore signals from other cells. These cancerous cells are called rogue cells.

- Cancer cells form in various sizes and are larger and darker than healthy cells, which are uniform in shape and size.

Tumor Development

Having one or more acquired risk factors and/or innate gene mutations, or variants, can damage cells, which, in turn, latch on to broken DNA. These cells solidify and formulate tumors that can lead to malignancy. (See front cover image).

However, all tumors are not cancerous; they can be benign, which means that they are non-cancerous and do not invade organ systems or other cells. Solid tumors, however, can be danger-ous if their size is so large that they put pressure on organs, blood vessels, or nerves.

"Liquid" cancer is another type of malignant tumor also made by cells. These cancerous tumors affect bone marrow, blood, lymph glands as well as the lymphatic system.

You can find information about the stages of cancer in the appendix.

The Perpetual Fight

Despite billions of dollars expended on curing cancer, a leading cause of death, the fight is still on. More than ten million people worldwide die annually from cancer, according to the World Health Organization.

According to the U.S. National Institutes of Health, an estimated 609,820 individuals will die from cancer in 2023 in the United States. Moreover, approximately 1,958,310 new cases of cancer will develop annually in the United States!

From 2016–2018, there were 375,400 new cancer cases in the United Kingdom. During that same timeframe 167,142 succumbed to the disease. Although somewhat dated, these figures, based on trends, are expected to rise.

What greatly bothers me is that after centuries and decades of fighting the fight against cancer, incidences of the dreaded disease continue to be prevalent. Over six decades ago, the National

Cancer Act of 1971 was signed into U.S. law. This law was intended to create U.S. clinical trial networks and lead to critical research in the care and treatment of cancer patients. Over a half century later, cancer still has *no real cure* despite millions of people and billions of dollars dedicated to curing cancer, many through charitable organizations.

Why is the cancer fight still being fought? It makes little sense to me. Although the research world understands the behavior of cancer cells, most cancers are yet to be cured. As Margaret I. Cuomo, M.D. stated in her 2012 book, *A World Without Cancer*, we need to take action to find a cure.

Fast forward eleven years since the publication of Dr. Cuomo's enlightening book, and we still have limited progress in preventing and curing cancer. For example, authors of a 2023 study, conducted at the Vanderbilt University Medical Center, discovered an anomaly regarding the immune system's T-cells. They found that the T-cells, which kill cancer cells or tumors, only are effective within a few hours of initial exposure to their specific antigens. These T-cells then became dysfunctional, leaving malignant tumors intact! This is an example of how research results continue to vary; one step forward, and two back.

Concluding Thoughts

This chapter presented an overview of a complex issue: cancer. Understanding vitamin D's mechanisms of action, I believe that *vitamin D deficiency* should be added to the list of cancer risk factors. The next chapter addresses how vitamin D regulates, *inter alia*, cell differentiation, cell proliferation, and natural cell death as well as other key cellular processes related to anti-cancer mechanisms of action.

6

ANTI-CANCER PROPERTIES

Vitamin D's extraordinary capability to prevent cancer is explored in this chapter. Some research also supports vitamin D aiding in the treatment of some early-stage cancers. This chapter explains vitamin D's mechanisms of action that have anti-cancer properties.

The *Defend Your Life* books describe several of vitamin D's mechanisms of action against the development of cancer. First and foremost, **you must enjoy an optimal vitamin D status to be effective in fighting cancer.** You may recall that your optimal vitamin D level should be at least 100 ng/mL or 250 nmol/L.

Let's address compelling vitamin D mechanisms of action that may decrease your risk of developing cancer. If interested, you can find molecular mechanisms of action in the "Geek Speak" boxes in this chapter.

- ***Acts as anti-inflammatory***: A fundamental advantage of supplementing with vitamin D and its two main cofactors (you can find this information in Chapter 13) is to decrease the incidences of inflammation. Optimal, activated vitamin D inhibits pro-inflammatory factors, which are derived from the risk factors stated in Chapter 5, and increases anti-inflammatory signals.

GEEK SPEAK

Vitamin D inhibits inflammation by *decreasing* COX-2 (cyclooxygenase 2), prostaglandin, stress kinase, and nuclear factor-$_k$B. In addition, it *increases* 15-PGDH (15-hydroxyprostaglandin dehydrogenase) and MAPKP5 (mitogen-activated protein kinase phosphatase 5).

- ***Protects against metastasis of cancer cells***: Patients diagnosed with cancer might ask, "Has the cancer spread or metastasized?" Optimal vitamin D levels have the capability to keep cancerous cells from spreading to tissue and healthy cells by decreasing signals that permit cancerous cells to penetrate through tissue and bind with other cells.

GEEK SPEAK

Vitamin D inhibits cancer cell invasion and metastasis by *decreasing* MMP-9 (matrix metalloproteinase 9), α6- and β4-integrins, as well as plasminogen activators. This process also *increases* TIMP-1 (tissue inhibitor of metalloproteinases 1) and E-cadherin.

- ***Prevents new blood vessels from forming that could support cancer***: Another advantage of having an optimal vitamin D status entails prevention of new blood cells from feeding cancerous cells. This mechanism of action disables the signals required to develop new blood vessels that could foster cancer cell development.

> **GEEK SPEAK**
>
> Vitamin D inhibits the development of new blood vessels by *decreasing* both VEGF (vascular endothelial growth factor) and HIF1-α (hypoxia inducible factor 1-α).

- ***Increases cell maturation (differentiation)***: Vitamin D increases cell-specific maturation and specialization. If cells remain immature, they are available to go rogue and transform into cancerous cells.

> **GEEK SPEAK**
>
> Vitamin D enhances the likelihood of differentiation of healthy cells by *increasing* differentiation factors such as casein, lipids, PSA (prostate-specific antigen), and E-cadherin.

- ***Inhibits Cell Proliferation***: Vitamin D halts uncontrolled cell reproduction that could lead to rogue cancer cells. Vitamin D also prevents chemical signals that are required for cells to divide.

GEEK SPEAK

Vitamin D inhibits cell proliferation by *decreasing* IGF-1 (insulin-like growth factor-1) and *increasing* IGF-1 binding protein and TGF-β (tumor necrosis factor β). In addition, vitamin D arrests the cell cycle by *increasing* p21 and p27 (cell cycle checkpoints), and *decreasing* CDKs, cyclins, MYC (proto-oncogene), and RB (tumor-suppressor protein).

- ***Promotes Apoptosis***: An integral function of healthy cells includes these cells dying a natural death, a process called apoptosis. Cells that will not die can proliferate into cancer cells. Vitamin D activates a process whereby broken-down cells are grouped into small packets, which are disposed of by innate immune cells called phagocytes.

GEEK SPEAK

Vitamin D promotes natural cell death, which activates internal apoptosis pathways by *increasing* BAX (pro-apoptotic protein) and *decreasing* BCL-2 (apoptosis regulating protein).

Concluding Thoughts

Well, there you have it: compelling vitamin D mechanisms of action that effectively prevent healthy cells from becoming cancerous cells. *Stop cancer before it begins—with optimal vitamin D!*

NOTE #1: If you are a member of Meta Facebook's "Vitamin D Wellness" Group and/or follow me on Facebook or X, you may recall a photo of a two-volume, blue tome on vitamin D research sitting next to the original *Defend Your Life* paperback book, challenging interested readers about which book would be easier to read? The information in the complementary tome contributed to the information in this chapter. The citation is listed in the Bibliography section.

NOTE #2: Within these chapters are "Geek Speak" information boxes that list *some* common DNA gene mutations, or variants, associated with selected types of cancer. These inherited gene variants are linked to increased risk of cancer. If your body has any of these gene variants, consider reducing cancer-related risks. Moreover, talk to a medical professional who understands genetic mutations. In addition, my book entitled *Silent Inheritance* explains some gene variants, genetic testing, etc.

7

VITAMIN D AND BREAST CANCER

One generally does not need a calendar to know when the month of October begins. We are simply inundated with the color pink, reminding us that it is Breast Cancer Awareness Month. Why, after several decades of recognizing Breast Cancer Awareness Month and pouring billions of dollars into medical research, does breast cancer remain the most common cancer among women in the world?

Sobering Statistics

One in eight women will be diagnosed with breast cancer in her lifetime, according to the American Cancer Society. Despite the unfathomable amount of money expended on breast cancer research, this statistic remains stable!

Globally, an estimated 2,261,419 new cases of breast cancer were diagnosed in 2020. The prevalence of breast cancer diagnoses is more than any other type of cancer. The median age of breast cancer diagnosis is age 63.

In 2023, approximately 297,790 women in the United States will be diagnosed with invasive breast cancer. In addition, about 55,720 will be diagnosed with *in situ* (non-invasive) breast cancer. For the past two decades invasive breast cancer cases have *increased* about one-half of a percent each year!

Let's not forget that men also can develop breast cancer. An estimated 2,800 males in the United States will be diagnosed with invasive breast cancer in 2023.

Female breast cancer worldwide is the fifth leading cause of death. The American Cancer Society projected that 43,700 persons (including 530 males) persons would die from breast cancer in the United States in 2023.

Notwithstanding these estimated death

statistics, survival from breast cancer is possible. If invasive cancer is only in the breast, the five-year survival rate of females with this disease is 99 percent. If the cancer has spread to the regional lymph nodes, the five-year survival rate is 86 percent. When breast cancer metastasizes, the survival rate is only 30 percent.

Actor-comedian-turned health writer Suzanne Somers passed away in October 2023, just before her 77th birthday, after a long battle with breast cancer. As she was an inspiration to me to speak out about vitamin D's benefits, I dedicate this chapter to Suzanne.

Vitamin D and Breast Cancer

I encourage you to rise above the "pink" not only in October but year around. In lieu of expensive diagnostic equipment and debilitating cancer drugs, why not consider the anti-cancer nutrient called vitamin D?

Research over the past several decades indicates that vitamin D plays an essential role in regulating cellular activity. Trillions of our cells contain vitamin D receptors (VDR) that receive, store, and, in many cases, produce vitamin D. These vitamin D anti-cancer functions, as we learned in the previous chapter, possess the capability to prevent cancer.

Vitamin D May Prevent Breast Cancer

Scientific research suggests that optimal vitamin D supplementation may prevent the onset of breast cancer:

- Canadian researchers studied the association of vitamin D levels with breast tumor size (non-metastatic). The circulating vitamin D levels of four hundred and seventy-six pre- and post-menopausal females were compared to breast cancer tumor size (Tumor grading is addressed in the appendix to this book). The research team concluded that females with "sufficient vitamin D levels at breast cancer diagnosis had smaller and lower grade tumors compared to women with insufficient vitamin D, especially among premenopausal women." They asserted that "maintaining optimal vitamin D levels in premenopausal women could improve prognostically important breast cancer characteristics at diagnosis." This study was published in the August 2023 issue of the journal *Clinical Breast Cancer.*

GEEK SPEAK

An Irish research team discovered that one of vitamin D's nutrient partners called vitamin K2 MK-4, or menaquinone-4, may *treat* two of the deadliest types of breast cancer: TNBC (triple-negative breast cancer) and HER2+ (human epidermal growth factor receptor). The study was published in the August 2015 issue of the journal *Nutritional Research*.

Vitamin D May Treat Breast Cancer

Research has suggested for some time that optimal vitamin D may help treat breast cancer.

- Egyptian scientists studied 221 hospital patients, who were an average age of 50.7 years, to ascertain vitamin D's association with advanced-stage breast cancer. The scientific team concluded that low circulating vitamin D is associated with advanced-stage breast cancer. Low vitamin D was more prevalent in HER2+ and TNBC patients. Furthermore, vitamin D had a "significant correlation with disease-free survival as well as overall survival." This study was reported in the August 2023 issue of the journal *Cancer Epidemiology*.

GEEK SPEAK

DNA gene mutations associated with <u>female</u> breast cancer *risk* factors include:

ATM	CHEK2
BARD1	CDH1
BRCA1	PALB2
BRCA2	RAD51D
PTEN	RAD51C
STK113	TP53

GEEK SPEAK

DNA gene mutations associated with <u>male</u> breast cancer *risk* factors include:

BRCA1	BRCA2
CHEK2	PALB2

Concluding Thoughts

Reflecting on breast cancer's sobering statistics, I cannot emphasize enough that optimal vitamin D3 supplementation may significantly reduce the risk of developing breast cancer. *Stop cancer before it begins—with optimal vitamin D!*

Furthermore, compelling research indicates that vitamin D may treat early stages of breast cancer.

In the next chapter let's look at vitamin D's effect on preventing and treating colorectal cancer.

8

VITAMIN D AND COLORECTAL CANCER

Colorectal cancer, commonly referred to as colon (large intestine) cancer, often is a silent killer unless you undergo regular diagnostic screenings. Cancers of the colon and rectum are the third-most common types of cancer in both men and women in the United States. Of course, vitamin D plays a big role in preventing and treating early-onset colorectal cancer, which is addressed later in this chapter.

Colorectal Cancer Statistics

Let's get an idea of how pervasive this cancer is throughout the world. As in the United States, colorectal cancer is the third most common cancer worldwide.

In 2023, approximately 153,020 adults in the United States were newly diagnosed with colon cancer. An estimated 1,880,725 persons around the world were diagnosed with colorectal cancer during 2020. Of this figure rectal cancer cases were about 732,210. (Please note that "colorectal" is a commonly used word to describe cancer in the colon and/or the rectum." Both "colon" and "rectum" cancer are frequently used together as they share similar features. Colon cancer begins in the colon, whereas rectal cancer starts in the rectum.)

The five-year survival rate for colorectal cancer in the U.S. is 65 percent.

Younger Adults Can Develop Colorectal Cancer

For decades, colorectal cancer was believed to occur primarily in people 50 years of age or older. In fact, public health campaigns strongly encourage people to undergo a colonoscopy when they turn 50. Many people heeded their advice, and subsequently, the incidence rate decreased in older adults in part due to the colonoscopies.

Surprisingly, colorectal cancer incidence has increased in younger adults. For example, if you were born between 1981 and 1996, you have twice the risk of colorectal cancer than people born in 1950. Furthermore, one-third of rectal cancer patients are under the age of 56 when diagnosed, and they are 60 percent more likely to have developed a more advanced form of the disease. For example, many younger people reportedly have severe gastrointestinal symptoms, e.g., rectal bleeding, persistent diarrhea, and abdominal pain, three months to two years prior to diagnosis. Having any one of these symptoms can double the risk of developing colorectal cancer.

Colorectal Polyps

Colorectal cancer usually develops as a non-cancerous growth called a polyp on the inner lining of the colon or rectum. Polyps are detected by a colonoscopy, a diagnostic screening tool to ascertain the condition of the colon and rectum. In addition, at-home tests (which require a prescription) can detect the presence of polyps as well as indications of cancer.

Many polyps are benign but can become cancerous due to risk factors such as genetics and inflammation. Malignant polyps usually grow into the inner lining of the colon or rectum, facilitating the spread of cancer to lymph nodes, blood, or other organs.

Vitamin D May Prevent Colorectal Cancer

More than 95 percent of colorectal cancers, or adenocarcinomas, start in the mucosal cells, which lubricate the lining of the colon and the rectum.

The mucosal cells contain vitamin D receptors (VDR) that receive and produce activated vitamin D. The VDR may protect against the risk factors stated in Chapter 5.

A plethora of research has been conducted on vitamin D and colorectal cancer over the past couple decades. Recent studies indicate vitamin D's positive effect on preventing colorectal cancer.

- Published in 2023 in the *International Journal of Cancer*, a report from a team of Chinese scientists described how higher levels of 25(OH)D were correlated with lower incidences of colon cancer. The scientists concluded their report by stating that vitamin D offers "potential benefits of maintaining optimal vitamin D for colorectal cancer prevention."

- An Italian research team examined the preventive role of vitamin D in colorectal cancer. Citing vitamin D's role in the immune system and gut microbial actions, the scientists were hopeful that additional studies would be conducted at the clinical level. The study was published in a 2022 issue of the journal *BioFactors*.

Vitamin D May Treat Early-stage Colorectal Cancer

Vitamin D receptors (VDR) in colon and rectum cells receive and produce activated vitamin D. By undertaking this process, vitamin D's mechanisms of action as stated in Chapter 6 have the potential to treat at least early-stages (stages 0 and 1) of colorectal cancer.

- Japanese researchers studied the risk of death or recurrences of digestive (includes colon and rectal) cancers in patients. The study was a randomized, double-blind, placebo-controlled clinical trial. The research team assessed that vitamin D supplementation of 2,000 IU daily reduced the risk of relapse or death in the digestive tract patients who possessed a mutated p53 gene. The results of the clinical trial were published in a 2023 issue of *JAMA Network Open*.

- According to Grassroots Health, esteemed vitamin D expert Dr. Michael Holick (who I have met) characterized the findings from this study as follows: "…*now proves beyond a doubt the power of vitamin D against cancer recurrence and fatality at the clinical level.*"

- A Chinese study, published in a 2021 edition of the *International Journal of Cancer*, evaluated the association between vitamin D status and colorectal cancer risk and survival. Using data from the UK Biobank, the research team researched 360,061 participants, 2,509 of whom were colorectal cancer survivors. The Chinese researchers found that higher concentrations of circulating vitamin D are not only connected to a lower incidence of colorectal cancer but also an improved *survival* from the disease.

GEEK SPEAK

DNA gene mutations associated with colorectal cancer *risk* factors include:

APC	CHEK2	p53
EPCAM	MLH2	MLH1
PMS2	PTEN	STK11
TP53	MUTYH	

Concluding Thoughts

Understanding how Chapter 6's vitamin D mechanisms of action mitigate cancer development, I believe that the association between vitamin D and colon and rectum cancers is real. However, additional trials at the clinical level should be conducted to ascertain the extent of how optimal vitamin D may contribute definitively to early-stage colon and rectum cancer survival.

Stop cancer before it begins—with optimal vitamin D!

The next chapter explains the connection between vitamin D and lung cancer.

9

VITAMIN D AND LUNG CANCER

Lung cancer is not caused only by tobacco smoke. Non-smokers, especially females, can also develop lung cancer. My dear cousin Patsy succumbed to lung cancer in her mid-fifties. Patsy, a non-smoker, endured interminable pain and suffering as a lung cancer patient. I dedicate this chapter to Patsy.

The most common form of lung cancer is non-small cell lung cancer (NSCLC). The second most prevalent type of lung cancer is referred to as small cell lung cancer (SCLC). Approximately 81 percent of all detected lung cancers incidences are diagnosed as NSCLC.

Lung Cancer Statistics

Lung cancer is the leading cause of cancer death for males and females across the globe. In 2020, about 1,796,144 people died globally from lung cancer. Also in 2020, an estimated 2,206,771 people worldwide were diagnosed with lung cancer. This figure includes both SCLC and NSCLC.

In 2023, an estimated 238,340 adults in the United States would be diagnosed with lung cancer, according to the American Cancer Society. This sobering figure comprised 120,790 females and 117,550 males, indicating that slightly more women are diagnosed with lung cancer than men.

As aging is one of the cancer risk factors, the incidence of lung cancer indeed increases with age. About 83 percent of lung cancer cases are diagnosed in persons aged 65 or older. Most cases of women with NSCLC are detected between the ages of 75 and 79. Whereas, men are most likely to be diagnosed with NSCLC between the ages of 80 and 84.

For people with non-spreading NSCLC, the general survival rate is about 65 percent. Unfortunately, about 70 percent of NSCLC people are diagnosed after the cancer has spread to the lymph nodes. When lung cancer metastasizes, the five-year survival rate is only 9 percent.

Primary Types of Lung Cancer

Non-small cell lung cancer (NSCLC) is the most commonly occurring type of lung cancer, according to the American Cancer Society. NSCLC forms in lung cells that produce mucus.

On the one hand, NSCLC is the most prevalent among people who never smoked, or *inter alia* young people. These patients' demographics point to gene mutations that are not inherited. The DNA gene variants connected to environmental risk factors are listed in the "Geek Speak" box.

On the other hand, SCLC is almost always caused by smoking. SCLC begins in cells around the bronchial airways. The cells appear round and small and spread quickly. In the United States the 5-year SCLC survival rate is 8 percent in women, and 6 percent in men.

GEEK SPEAK

DNA gene mutations associated with lung cancer *risk* factors include:

ALK   EGFR
KRAS   ROS1

Vitamin D May Prevent Lung Cancer

At the time of this writing, I am unaware of recent science that specifically addresses prevention of lung cancer. Suffice to say, the anti-cancer mechanisms of action addressed in Chapter 6 most likely may prevent the development of lung cancer in at least in low-risk persons.

Vitamin D May Treat Early-stage Lung Cancer

The VDR in lung cells receive and produce activated vitamin D. By undertaking this process, vitamin D's anti-cancer properties possess the means to treat at least early-onset (stages 0 and 1) lung cancer.

- A research paper, published in the February 2021 issue of the journal *Gene*, investigated the effect vitamin D had on *in vitro* malignant tumor cells in mice. The researchers concluded that vitamin D inhibits the proliferation, invasion, and metastasis of NSCLC as well as promotes apoptosis (natural cell death). ***

- Chinese researchers studied vitamin D's behavior regarding the downregulation of a protein called "histidine-rich calcium-bonding protein" (HRC) in relation to the limitation of lung cancer cells. The scientists concluded that "vitamin D inhibited lung cancer tumor growth, migration, and proliferation by downgrading HRC" in mice. The takeaway from the study is that vitamin D's anti-cancer effects, once again, were demonstrated in this study, which was published in a 2021 issue of the *Journal of Advanced Research*.

*** Note to my readers: In preparation for writing a *Defend Your Life* book, I research the medical literature to ascertain the science about vitamin D's role in a specific topic. My general policy is to cite only research that used human beings (*in* *vivo*) as subjects. Unfortunately, these two afore-mentioned studies used mice (*in vitro*) as research subjects. The dearth of human research during the beginning of the 2020 decade may have been due to staffing issues during the COVID-19 pandemic. ✳✳✳

- Japanese researchers conducted a random-ized, double-blind, placebo-controlled trial to examine whether vitamin D3 supplementation (1,200 IU daily) can improve the prognosis of patients with NSCLC. The study revealed that vitamin D3 supplementation, even at a relatively low dose, improves survival from lung cancer. The study was published in a September 2018 issue of the journal *Clinical Cancer Research*.

Concluding Thoughts

Vitamin D's anti-cancer properties are noteworthy in preventing lung cancers and treating early-stage (0 and 1) lung cancers. I hope you have a better understanding of lung cancer, its survival rate, risk factors, and vitamin D's protective effects. *Stop cancer before it begins—with optimal vitamin D!*

10

VITAMIN D AND PANCREATIC CANCER

I wrote about pancreatic cancer because it has an extremely low survival rate. I have also noted that the incidence of persons perishing from pancreatic cancer has risen. In fact, the often-fatal disease is rising rapidly in persons younger than the age of 55, as well as a higher incidence in males than females. And it is common for pancreatic cancer to go undetected until it is too late.

Understanding vitamin D's therapeutic effect on many cancers, I challenged myself to research medical literature that suggests how vitamin D can prevent pancreatic cancer.

First, let's look at some sobering statistics about this type of cancer. Then we will take a brief look at the pancreas and how cancer forms in that organ.

Stunning Statistics

Pancreatic cancer is often fatal, according to the American Cancer Society's (ACS) statistics. The ACS estimated that 64,050 people would be diagnosed with pancreatic cancer in the United States in 2023.

More than 50,000 people in the United States would die of pancreatic cancer in 2023. This often-deadly cancer accounts for approximately seven percent of all cancer deaths worldwide. The survival rate of Stage 4 pancreatic cancer is about one percent.

The average lifetime risk of pancreatic cancer is about 1 in 64. Of course, the severity of the risk factors affects the chances of developing this cruel disease.

Pancreas Basics

The pancreas is an organ nestled behind the stomach; its neighbors include the small intestine, spleen, gallbladder, and liver. We cannot live well without a functional pancreas as it is vital to both the digestive and endocrine systems.

Major types of cells in the pancreas include *exocrine* and *endocrine.* The latter (about five percent of the pancreatic cells) produce insulin and other chemicals that are released directly into the bloodstream. On the other hand, exocrine cells in the pancreas produce chemical messengers that help digest food. (Pancreatic cancer develops when exocrine cells begin proliferating in the ducts of this gland).

GEEK SPEAK

DNA gene mutations associated with pancreatic cancer *risk* factors include:

ATM	**CDKN2A**
BRCA1*	**MLH1**
BRCA2*	**PALB2**

***You may think that BRCA1 and BRCA2 gene variants are only associated with breast cancer in females and males but that is not the case. BRCA1 and BRCA2 gene mutations are also connected, *inter alia,* to skin cancer (melanoma), cancer of female reproductive organs, and prostate cancer.**

Vitamin D May Help Prevent Cancer

At the time of this writing, I am unaware of any studies that specifically address prevention of pancreatic cancer. Suffice it to say, the anti-cancer mechanisms of action addressed in Chapter 6 most likely may prevent the development of pancreatic cancer in low-risk persons.

Vitamin D May Treat Early-stage Pancreatic Cancer

A 2018 U.S. review of vitamin D's role in treating pancreatic cancer led to several clinical trials including the two cited below. As a result of this review, researchers found that vitamin D's potent effect on the immune system combined with oncolytic virotherapy, which eventually leads to cancer cell death without harming healthy cells.

Recent clinical trials are designed to explain how optimal vitamin D may have a therapeutic effect on patients with pancreatic cancer.

- An objective of an active clinical trial, sponsored by the Dana-Farber Cancer Institute, was to ascertain the effect of paricalcitol (a synthetic form of vitamin D) and other chemicals on treating metastatic pancreatic adenocarcinoma. The trial would be scheduled to be completed by November 2025.

- Sponsored by Emory University in collaboration with the U.S. National Cancer Institute, the second phase of a clinical trial (which was recruiting subjects in March 2023) was planned. This clinical trial would investigate how well paricalcitol, which inhibits the growth and spread of a malignant tumor, and hydroxychloroquine, which denies cancer cells to use energy to grow, work in tandem to treat metastasized pancreatic cancer.

Concluding Thoughts

I am encouraged that the scientific community recognizes at least some vitamin D benefits in treating pancreatic cancer. Clinical trials should provide useful data to explore further vitamin D therapies.

Regarding prevention, I, once again, exclaim, *"Stop cancer before it begins—with optimal vitamin D!"* Maintaining optimal vitamin D levels as well as leading a healthy lifestyle may go a long way to decreasing the risk of pancreatic cancer.

The next chapter addresses vitamin D's positive effect on the prevention and treatment of prostate cancer.

11

VITAMIN D AND PROSTATE CANCER

Prostate cancer is another silent and sometimes lethal disease. Cancer of the prostate—a male reproductive organ—is the second-leading cause of male cancer deaths in the United States. (Skin cancer is the leading cause of death in males. You can find information about skin cancer in the next chapter.)

Prostate Cancer Statistics

In 2020, about 375,304 men worldwide died from prostate cancer. According to the American Cancer Society, an estimated 34,700 deaths from prostate cancer would be projected to occur in the United States in 2023.

Despite improved screening procedures, overall incidences of prostate cancer have increased by about three percent each year. Unfortunately, cases of advanced-stage prostate cancer increased by five percent in 2020.

Estimated prostate cancer incidences in 2023 were about 288,300 persons in the United States. In 2020, about 1,414,259 people were diagnosed worldwide.

An encouraging statistic is that prostate cancer's five-year survival rate is about 97 percent. Nonetheless, prostate cancer can be serious; if the cancer has spread to other parts of the body, the five-year survival rate is only 32 percent.

Prostate-specific Antigen (PSA)

The prostate gland secretes a substance called prostate-specific antigen or PSA. Testing a patient's blood serum for PSA can indicate the presence or absence of prostate cancer. An elevated level of

PSA (>10ng/mL), like some other cancers, can be affected by risk factors including genetics, aging, or dietary factors (you can find overall cancer risk factors in Chapter 5).

NOTE: Within these chapters are "Geek Speak" information boxes that list *some* common DNA gene mutations, or variants, associated with selected types of cancer. These inherited gene variants are linked to increased risk of cancer. If your body has any of these gene variants, consider reducing cancer-related risks. Moreover, talk to a medical professional who understands genetic mutations. In addition, my book entitled *Silent Inheritance* explains some gene variants, genetic testing, etc.

GEEK SPEAK

DNA gene mutations associated with prostate cancer *risk* factors include:

ATM	**CHEK1**
BRCA1	**HOXB13**
BRCA2	**PALB2**

Vitamin D May Prevent Prostate Cancer

In addition to a plethora of medical research published over the past couple decades, recent studies continue to indicate vitamin D's positive effect on preventing prostate cancer.

- Published in a 2023 issue of the *European Journal of Cancer*, a study, conducted by scientists from the German Cancer Research Center in Heidelberg, examined the association of vitamin D status and mortality due to, *inter alia*, prostate cancer. The research team concluded that low vitamin D is associated with an increased chance of death from prostate and other cancers.

- A review reported in an April 2023 issue of the *Journal of Steroid Biochemistry and Molecular Biology* focused on the impact of vitamin D on cancer including prostate cancer. The researchers concluded that "significant progress in understanding the multiple roles that vitamin D plays in our bodies" suggests "the anti-cancer properties of vitamin D may have a long-term impact on human lives as we age and succumb to injuries and disease."

Vitamin D May Treat Early-stage Prostate Cancer

Vitamin D receptors (VDR) in prostate gland cells receive and produce activated vitamin D. By undertaking this process, vitamin D has the potential to treat at least early stages of prostate cancer.

At the time of this writing, there is little *recent* information about vitamin D and prostate cancer treatment. Nonetheless, researchers of a randomized clinical trial of U.S. military veterans that was conducted in 2012-2015 and *updated in June 2020,* hypothesized that only 4,000 IU daily vitamin D3 supplementation would decrease the likelihood of undergoing radiation therapy or a prostatectomy.

Concluding Thoughts

Although its mortality rate is less than many other cancers, prostate cancer should be taken seriously. Optimal vitamin D status decreases the risk of developing prostate cancer as well as treating the early stages of the disease. *Stop cancer before it begins—with optimal vitamin D!*

The next chapter addresses vitamin D and skin cancer including melanoma.

12

VITAMIN D AND SKIN CANCER

Writing about vitamin D, the sunshine vitamin, and skin cancer is a bit tricky. On the one hand, sunlight can make vitamin D in the skin, our largest organ. On the other hand, significant exposure to sunlight can cause skin cancers including melanoma, potentially lethal skin cancer!

So, what can we do? We can only have a conservatively moderate dose of UVB sunlight on our bare skin. If we must be out in the sun, then we need to dress accordingly, stay in the shade whenever possible, and my least favorite option: apply sunscreen (chemicals) for the skin. Before we delve into these thoughts, let's take a brief look at the four major types of lesions that are associated with skin cancer.

Types of Skin Cancer

Pre-cancer lesions, or actinic keratosis, are highly common and usually are monitored closely for change in characteristics, e.g., color, size, and shape. It is not unusual for pre-cancerous lesions to be removed by a dermatologist.

Basal cell carcinoma, a non-melanoma cancer, is the most common skin cancer; it accounts for more than 90 percent of all types of skin cancer. Basal cell carcinoma typically is slow-growing and usually does not spread to other parts of the body.

Squamous cell carcinoma is a non-melanoma cancer that is more likely than basal cell carcinoma to spread to other organs, if left undiagnosed and excised.

Melanoma is a potentially deadly skin cancer because it can spread into the bloodstream, lymphatic system, and organs. Melanoma can develop <u>anywhere</u> on the body including under fingernails, between toes, etc. This cancer begins in cells that produce melanin (skin color) called *melanocytes*.

Melanomas are challenging to diagnose as they do not always begin as a mole and can appear as normal-looking skin. The way to diagnose melanoma is for a dermatologist to surgically excise the "mole" or lesion and send it to a laboratory for analysis. Depending upon the laboratory results, Mohs surgery could be necessary to ensure that all melanoma has been removed from the site.

MERKEL CELL CARCINOMA

In September 2023, beloved American singer Jimmy Buffett succumbed to a form of a little-known skin cancer called Merkel cell carcinoma. He suffered from the disease for four years until his death.

Although Merkel cell carcinoma is rare, it is the second most common cause of skin cancer *death* after melanoma. Merkel grows and spreads quickly, but research to better understand the disease is still limited.

Males are two times more likely than females to develop Merkel.

The Centers for Disease Control and Prevention (CDC) suggest that a strong immune system may help to prevent cancer as well as other protective measures to thwart skin cancers. The book *Defend Your Life III* is devoted to vitamin D's positive impact on the immune system.

Melanoma Statistics

In 2020, skin cancers were the most common group of cancers diagnosed in the world with 1.5 million new cases of melanoma. Globally, about 57,000 people died from melanoma during that same year. In 2023, an estimated 7,990 people in the United States would succumb to melanoma. In the U.S. melanoma accounts for about one percent of all skin cancers. However, it causes the majority of skin cancer deaths.

Association between Vitamin D and Melanoma

Recent research about the association between vitamin D supplementation and melanoma includes:

- A Finnish cross-sectional study of 498 adults concluded that regular use of a vitamin D supplement is connected to fewer melanoma patients compared to those subjects who did not take vitamin D supplements. The study was published in the 1 April 2023 issue of the journal *Melanoma Research*.

SUE'S STORY: In my mid-twenties, I was diagnosed with melanoma by my doctor, who noticed an irregularly shaped, dark mole on my upper right arm. At that age, I had only vaguely heard of vitamin D as "the sunshine vitamin." I knew nothing else about this vitamin.

Subsequently, the melanoma lesion was surgically excised down to, but not including, the muscle. In addition, a significant perimeter of skin in the area was removed. The surgical site was covered with a skin graft from my upper thigh. The healing process was painful for years. To this day I sport a large gap in my upper right arm.

So, why did I develop melanoma? I believe the cancer was caused by a lot of sunbathing, i.e., direct, UVA light exposure, without protection as well as incurring sun poisoning a couple of times as a teenager.

The lesson learned is that we should not be in direct sunlight longer than 15-20 minutes before covering ourselves with appropriate clothing and sunscreen. By doing so, the risk of developing melanoma (and the other types of skin cancer) will decrease.

- Researchers from Spain and Chile studied 286 stages 1 and 2 melanoma patients whose circulating vitamin D levels were measured at the time of diagnosis. They concluded that circulating vitamin D levels less than 9.25 ng/mL are associated with melanoma development in the surface of the skin. As you know by reading Part I of this book, a value of 9.25 ng/mL is barely traceable. In other words, low levels of serum vitamin D most likely will influence the development of cutaneous melanoma. The study was published in a 2022 issue of the journal *ACTAS Dermo-Sifiliograficas*.

- Reported in a 2021 issue of the journal *Nutrients*, Spanish researchers addressed "practical" recommendations regarding the association between vitamin D and skin cancer. The authors admitted that there were no widely applicable strategies to prevent skin cancer. However, melanoma patients, as well as people who are at risk of cutaneous cancer, should have their serum vitamin D periodically monitored.

GEEK SPEAK

DNA gene mutations associated with melanoma *risk* factors include:

BAP1	BRCA1
BRCA2	CDK4
CDKN2A	PTEN
TP53	

Concluding Thoughts

Many of us are likely to develop some form of skin cancer from excessive exposure to ultraviolet A and B rays, both naturally from the sun as well as indoor tanning.

Skin carcinomas usually lie quietly for years or decades until a weakened immune system unleashes cancer cells. Acquiring and maintaining an optimal vitamin D level is one way to bolster your immune system. Get regular (at least annual) checkups with a dermatologist. Wear protective clothing and stay in the shade when outdoors.

Stop cancer before it begins—with an optimal vitamin D level! Speaking of which, the next part tells you how to easily raise your vitamin D level to one that is ideal, thus providing potential protection against cancer. Part III also presents the popular Vitamin D Wellness Protocol, accessed by over fifty thousand members in the Meta Facebook "Vitamin D Wellness" Group.

Raise Your Vitamin D

13

THE VITAMIN D WELLNESS PROTOCOL

Due to our modern lifestyles and conventional medical practices, we tend to get little vitamin D from its natural source, ultraviolet B, or UVB, sun rays. From living, commuting, and working indoors to using sunscreen, we deny ourselves this essential nutrient. As most diets are severely lacking in vitamin D, the most practical way of getting optimal vitamin D is by taking an inexpensive daily, oral D3 supplement (as well as vitamin K2, and magnesium).

By following my daily Vitamin D Wellness Protocol, my vitamin D level has been more than optimal (greater than or equal to 100 ng/mL [250 nmol/L]) for years. The health benefits described in this book speak for themselves.

The Vitamin D Wellness Protocol

Tens of thousands of people have accessed the tri-nutrient Vitamin D Wellness Protocol via my website: smilinsuepubs.com and the Meta Facebook group called "Vitamin D Wellness." Here is the Protocol in a nutshell:

TAKE DAILY AFTER BREAKFAST:
10,000 to 20,000 IU VITAMIN D3
90-120 mcg VITAMIN K2 MK-7
400-600 mg MAGNESIUM MALATE

Vitamin D3: Most diets do not contain optimal vitamin D. Start by taking 5,000 IU *daily* of vitamin D3 oil-based (soft gels or liquid) supplements with or right after your breakfast. After the first week, take 10,000 IU a day. **Then take 20,000 IU each day after two weeks to increase**

your level. After achieving your optimal vitamin D status, maintain it by taking 10,000 IU daily. (Please note that people who have kidney or liver issues should consult their healthcare provider prior to taking vitamin D3.)

Vitamin K2: A vitamin K2 diet includes lots of grass-fed meat and dairy products. Since most of us are lacking a daily, abundant intake of grass-fed foods, supplement with about 100 mcg of non-soy vitamin K2 MK-7. Take your K2 and D3 together with, or right after, your breakfast, which should include healthy fats such as egg yolks, cottage cheese, other cheeses, avocado, and nuts.

Magnesium: Magnesium-rich foods include leafy green vegetables such as spinach, legumes, avocado, nuts, seeds, and dark chocolates. A *daily* supplement of magnesium malate of 400 to 600 mg should boost your levels of this essential mineral. Magnesium *malate* should be taken in the morning as it may promote energy.

IMPORTANT NOTES:
1) Please do not take any form of vitamin K if you are on blood-thinning medication without the approval of your health care practitioner. 2) If you are taking thyroid medication, avoid taking a *soy*-based product, e.g., natto. Soy may disrupt the

efficacy of thyroid hormone medication. An alternative to soy is vitamin K2 MK-7 that is derived from fermented chickpeas. 3) Persons taking thyroid medication should wait at least *four* hours before taking any magnesium or other mineral supplements.

CONCLUDING THOUGHTS

"*Stop Cancer Before It Begins—with Optimal Vitamin D!*" Yes, once again, I state my mantra. I hope that you seriously consider it and follow the daily Vitamin D Wellness Protocol.

Aim for an optimal D3 level of at least 100 ng/mL or 250 nmol/L. Get tested every six months until you have achieved your goal. Maintain your optimal D level by continuing to follow the Vitamin D Wellness Protocol but decrease your daily dose of vitamin D3 to 10,000 IU.

Vitamin D's extraordinary properties culminate, when activated by optimal vitamin D levels, as anti-cancer mechanisms of action in the immune system. They can prevent cancer initiation and growth if you acquire optimal vitamin D.

Remember that cancer is a genetic disease. Decrease your risk of getting cancer by considering how to counter environmental and genetic factors. For example, if you lead a sedentary lifestyle—get some regular exercise; if you smoke—quit, etc.

As I conclude writing *Defend Your Life V*, I sincerely hope you have found this book helpful and informative about how optimal vitamin D may reduce the risk of developing cancer. And, in some cases, optimal vitamin D may treat early-stages (0 and 1) of cancer.

Let vitamin D help you attain your health goals. Take care.

~ Sue

P.S. If you find *Defend Your Life V* informative, please consider sharing a positive rating or brief review on Amazon. Thank you.

APPENDIX

Cancer Staging

You probably have heard the word "stage" when describing the extent that cancer has grown and spread. For example, if you heard, "she was diagnosed with Stage 1 colon cancer," it would mean that the tumor has grown *into* the submucosa, which is the layer of tissue directly underneath the mucosa, or the lining of the colon.

Cancer staging is important for the diagnosis and treatment of cancer. Staging describes where the malignant tumor is located, its spread to the lymph nodes, and its effect on other parts of the body. The lowest concern for cancer is a zero, and the highest is a four, written as "stage 4" or "stage IV."

"Stage 0," means the cancer is non-invasive or *in situ*, and has been detected early in its potential progression. As a comparison, "Stage 4" cancer is highly invasive of regional lymph nodes and has spread to other organs.

A more detailed characterization of describing cancer stages is called the **TNM+G** system:

- "**T**" plus a number (from 0 to 4) that represents how much the *tumor* has grown into the organ walls.
- "**N**" plus a number or letter (from 0 to 4b) stands for *lymph nodes,* small organs located throughout the body. Lymph nodes are part of the immune system.
- "**M**" plus a number and letter (M0 to M1c) describes the extent cancer has *metastasized* (spread) to other parts of the body beyond the tumor site, such as the lungs or liver.
- "**G**" plus a number or letter (GX to G4) represents the *grade* of the tumor. It describes how much cancer cells look like healthy cells—a process called differentiation. For example, a grade of G3 indicates that cancer cells look less like healthy cells—the malignant cells are called "poorly differentiated."

For example, in a case of colon cancer, a doctor characterized a tumor as **T2 N1a M0 G2**. The *tumor* cells have grown into a deeper, thick layer of the muscle that helps to move along the contents of the intestines. The tumor cells are in one regional *lymph node;* they have not spread to two or more regional lymph nodes. The disease has not *metastasized* to a distant part of the body. The *grade* of the malignant cells refers to how they compare to healthy cells. The tumor cells are characterized as moderately differentiated.

ADDITIONAL RESOURCES

Books

Defend Your Life (2013) Introduction to Vitamin D. (Won an international Mom's Choice® Award.)

Silent Inheritance (2017): Understanding Depression. (DNA gene variants, etc.)

Defend Your Life II (2019) Vitamin D: Better Health from Preconception through Adulthood.

Defend Your Life III (2022) Vitamin D and Immunity.

Defend Your Life IV (2023) Vitamin D and Allergies (plus Asthma)

****All books are by Susan Rex Ryan. Paper and electronic copies are available via Amazon.*

Immune. Dettmer, Philipp. Random House. 2021. Hardcover and electronic copies are available via Amazon.

A World Without Cancer, Margaret I. Cuomo. Rodale.
    2012. Print, electronic, and audio versions are available via Amazon.

Websites

Website: www.smilinsuepubs.com. The author's website
    and blog.

Website: www.grassrootshealth.net. Vitamin D-related
    information.

In addition, vitamin D organizations can be found globally
    via an online search; these countries include Canada,
    Pakistan, and the United Kingdom.

BIBLIOGRAPHY

Akiba, Tadashi et al. "Vitamin D Supplementation and Survival of Patients with Non-small Cell Lung Cancer: A Randomized, Double-Blind, Placebo-Controlled Trial." *Clinical Cancer Research.* 2018 Sep 1;24(17):4089-4097.

Cuomo, Margaret I. *A World Without Cancer.* Rodale. 2012.

Dettmer, Philipp. *Immune.* Random House, 2021.

Editorial. "Cause for concern: the rising incidence of early-onset pancreatic cancer." *The Lancet Gastroenterology & Hepatology.* 2023 April;8:287.

Feldman, David et al. *Vitamin D: Third Edition, Volume 1.* Academic Press. 2011.

Kanasuo, Emilia et al. "Regular use of vitamin D supplement is associated with fewer melanoma cases compared to non-use: a cross-sectional study in 498 adult subjects at risk of skin cancers." *Melanoma Research.* 2023 April 1:33(2):126-135.

Kanno, Kazuki et al. "Effect of Vitamin D Supplements on Relapse or Death in p53-Immunoreactive Subgroup with Digestive Tract Cancer: Post Hoc Analysis of the AMATERASU Randomized Clinical Trial." *JAMA Network Open.* 2023;6(8):e2328886.

Kiely, Maeve et al. "Realtime cell analysis of the inhibitory effect of vitamin K2 on adhesion and proliferation of breast cancer cells." *Nutrition Research.* 2015 August;35(8):736-43.

LaRocca, Christopher J. and Warner, Susanne G. "A New Role for Vitamin D: The Enhancement of Oncolytic Viral Therapy in Pancreatic Cancer. *Biomedicines.* 2018 November 5;6:104.

Li, Jiaoyuan et al. "Serum vitamin D concentration, vitamin D-related polymorphisms, and colorectal cancer risk." *International Journal of Cancer.* 2023 July 15;153(2):278-289.

Lin, Hui-Yi et al. "Dietary and Serum Antioxidants Associated with Prostate-Specific Antigen for Middle-Aged and Older Men." *Nutrients.* 2023 July 25; 15:3298.

Liu, Ning et al. "Inhibition of lung cancer by vitamin D depends on downregulation of histidine-rich calcium-binding protein." *Journal of Advanced Research.* 2021:13-22.

Manocha, Amit et al. "Low Serum Vitamin D Associated with Increased Tumor Size and Higher Grade in Premenopausal Canadian Women with

Breast Cancer." *Clinical Breast Cancer.* 2023; August;23(6):e368-e376.

Martin-Gorgojo, Alejandro. "Vitamin D and Skin Cancer: An Epidemiological, Patient-Centered Update and Review." *Nutrients.* 2021 November 28;13:4292.

Mohamed, Rehab F. et al. "Low baseline vitamin D levels increase the risk of bone metastases among females with breast cancer – Hospital based cohort study." *Cancer Epidemiology.* 2023 August;85:102374.

Moro, R. et al. "Prognostic Value of Vitamin D Serum Levels in Cutaneous Melanoma." *ACTAS Dermo-Sifiliograficas.* 2022 March 4;113(T347-T353.

Rinninella, Emanuele et al. "Vitamin D and colorectal cancer: Chemopreventive perspectives through the gut microbiota and the immune system." *BioFactors.* 2022;48:285-293.

Seraphin, Gerbenn et al. "The impact of vitamin D on cancer: A mini review." *Journal of Steroid Biochemistry and Molecular Biology.* 2023 April 11;231:106308.

Sha Sha et al. "Associations of 25-hydroxyvitamin D status and vitamin D supplementation use with mortality due to 18 frequent cancer types in the UK Biobank cohort." *European Journal of Cancer.* 2023 July 17;191:113241.

Trump, Donald L. and Aragon-Ching, Jeanny. "Vitamin D in prostate cancer." *Asian Journal of Andrology.* 2018 May-June;20(3):244-252.

Xu, Gui-Ping et al. "The association between BRCA1 gene polymorphism and cancer risk: a meta-analysis." *Oncotarget.* 2018;9(9):8681-8694.

Zhou, Jian et al. "Associations of vitamin D status with colorectal cancer risk and survival." *International Journal of Cancer.* 2021 March 30;149(3):606-614.

GLOSSARY

1,25-dihydroxyvitamin D (1,25(OH)2D): a vitamin D test that measures activated vitamin D. This test is not recommended for reasons stated in Chapter 4.

7-dehydrocholesterol: a chemical produced in the skin when exposed to UVB rays.

25-hydroxyvitamin D (25(OH)D): the gold standard for testing circulating vitamin D or calcidiol.

ACS: American Cancer Society, headquartered in Atlanta, Georgia.

AMA: American Medical Association, headquartered in Chicago, Illinois.

Antibody: made by a type of white blood cell in response to an antigen.

Antigen: "a piece of an enemy that [your] immune system can recognize."

Antiserum: blood serum that contains antibodies against specific antigens.

B-Cell: an immune cell that slows down and neutralizes pathogens by producing antibodies.

Boron: a little-known element that partners with vitamin D.

CAC: a non-invasive test called "CT coronary artery calcium" scoring.

Calcidiol: circulating vitamin D in the blood.

Calcium: the most abundant mineral in the body that builds and maintains strong bones.

Calcitriol: activated vitamin D in the cells.

Casein: a protein found in milk.

CDC: The Centers for Disease Control and Prevention, headquartered in Atlanta, Georgia.

Cholecalciferol: vitamin D3.

COVID-19: the highly contagious coronavirus that caused a pandemic from early 2020 until 2022.

DNA: deoxyribonucleic acid is a molecule that contains genetic information. DNA comprises two linked strands wound around each other to resemble a twisted ladder—called the double helix.

EML: Essential Medicines List controlled by the WHO.

Endocrine: cells in the pancreas that produce insulin.

Ergocalciferol: vitamin D2, a less effective form of vitamin D.

Exocrine: cells in the pancreas that produce chemical messengers that aid in digestion.

FDA: U.S. Food and Drug Administration, headquartered in Silver Spring, Maryland.

Glucose: blood sugar.

Glycosides: chemicals used in some heart medications, e.g., digoxin.

HER2+: human epidermal growth factor receptor. One of the deadliest forms of breast cancer.

In situ: in place or position; undisturbed.

IU: international unit, a common form of measurement of vitamin D supplements.

Lymphocytes: "natural killer" white blood cells, such as B- and T-cells.

Macrophages: large white blood cells that fight pathogens.

Magnesium: a nutritional chemical element that partners with vitamin D.

Mast cell: a large cell that carries chemicals including histamine.

Melanin: skin color.

Melanocytes: cells where skin color begins (related to melanoma).

Melanoma: a potentially lethal skin cancer.

Menaquinone: vitamin K2.

Merkel: a rare lethal melanoma.

Mohs: precise and gradual skin surgery to avoid excising too much healthy skin.

Natto: fermented soybeans that are rich in vitamin K2 MK-7.

Neutrophils: front-line white blood cells that surround and capture pathogens.

NSCLC: non-small cell lung cancer.

Parathyroid: four tiny glands that help to regulate calcium levels by releasing parathyroid hormone or PTH. Parathyroid glands are located behind the thyroid gland.

Paricalcitol: a synthetic form of vitamin D used in some research.

Pathogen: any invader of the immune system that can cause an allergic reaction or illness.

Phagocytes: innate immune cells.

Phosphorus: a mineral (also referred to as phosphate) that interacts with vitamin D, calcium, and PTH.

Phylloquinone: vitamin K1.

Prostaglandin: a group of fat compounds.

Protein: a molecule that comprises amino acids, which are tiny organic building blocks, that are strung together like a chain.

PTH: parathyroid glands, nestled in the neck, that regulate calcium.

RBC Magnesium: a more accurate magnesium test than the serum magnesium blood test. The RBC version measures magnesium in red blood cells.

SCLC: small cell lung cancer.

Sunscreen: chemical substances designed to protect the skin by blocking the penetration of UVA and UVB rays.

T-Cell: an immune cell that targets and attacks a pathogen.

TNBC: triple-negative breast cancer.

Ultraviolet B (UVB) rays: invisible rays that come primarily from sunlight. A moderate exposure (15-20 minutes) around noon should initiate vitamin D production in the skin.

URTI: upper respiratory tract infection.

VDR: vitamin D receptors that are the proteins that allow the cells to receive activated vitamin D.

Vitamin A: a fat-soluble nutrient required in small quantities to support metabolism. Vitamin A also is a partner with vitamin D.

Vitamin K1: a vital, blood-clotting nutrient that is recycled in the body.

Vitamin K2: a vitamin D partner nutrient that facilitates moving calcium to the bones and teeth.

Vitamin K2 MK-4: a form of vitamin K2 that is found in grass-fed foods.

Vitamin K2 MK-7: a more effective form of vitamin K2 that is found in some soy products.

WHO: World Health Organization, headquartered in Geneva, Switzerland.

Zinc: an essential trace element that supports the immune system and is a cofactor of vitamin D.

ACKNOWLEDGMENTS

Defend Your Life V would not exist without the outstanding research that has been published on vitamin D and its association with cancer. I thank the scores of researchers and scientists who are as passionate about exploring vitamin D's role in human health as I am.

Thank you to organizations such as the American Cancer Society for their tireless work on cancer awareness and research.

I would like to thank the folks at Grassroots Health for providing insightful information about vitamin D's anti-cancer effects.

Special thanks to my husband Dave who reviewed my draft work to make it better for you, the reader.

The cover and interior design of *Defend Your Life V* are products of an outstanding graphic design professional named Shannon Bodie of BookWise Design in Oregon. The visual magic created by Shannon and her team accentuates the theme of this book.

Finally, much gratitude to the administrators of the Vitamin D Wellness support group on Meta Facebook. The admin team tirelessly responds to scores of daily questions and offers lots of support to over 55,000 members.

ABOUT THE AUTHOR

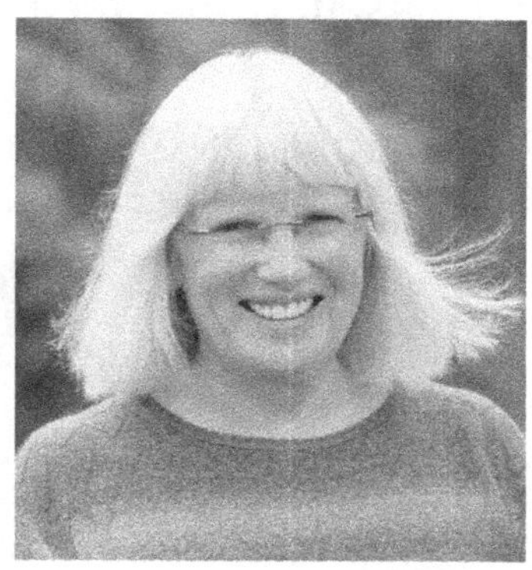

Susan "Sue" Rex Ryan was born and raised in Pennsylvania. She earned a Bachelor of Science degree at Georgetown University. Sue also holds a Master of Science degree from the U.S. military's National War College in Washington, D.C. She has earned scores of Continuing Medical Education, or CME, credits from accredited U.S. medical programs approved by, *inter alia*, The American Academy of Family Physicians.

Sue is the author of the popular *Defend Your Life* Vitamin D health books. Her debut book won a prestigious Mom's Choice Award®, an international award program that recognizes authors and others for their efforts in creating quality, family-friendly media products.

Although not submitted for award consideration, *Defend Your Life II* won the hearts of readers for its focus on life itself, from preconception through adulthood.

In 2022, *Defend Your Life III* won an international Firebird Book Award for the best health book in its category. This book addresses vitamin D's benefits to prevent and treat contagious, upper respiratory infections.

Defend Your Life IV was published in 2023 to convey the association between vitamin D and allergies.

Sue and her husband Dave reside in the sunny suburbs of Las Vegas, Nevada. They enjoy traveling to visit family and friends, as well as experiencing various cultures in Argentina, Easter Island, French Polynesia, Peru, Qatar, and Sri Lanka.

Sue welcomes your visit to her website "smilinsuepubs.com" that is replete with her blog articles about health topics. You can also follow her on social media including Meta Facebook and X @VitD3Sue.